CONQUER THYSELF

Everything I Need to Remember
To Maintain Total Well-Being

D. A. Metrov

DEDICATION

To my beloved wife, Maureen, without whom this book may have never been written. And our cat who reminds me to nap often.

Thank you for reading!
If you enjoy this book, you can learn more about the author and his other books at www.lightmasters.net.
Your review on Amazon.com would be most welcome.

IMPORTANT:

Neither the publisher nor the author is engaged in rendering professional advice or services to the individual reader. The ideas, procedures, and suggestions in this book are not intended as a substitute for consulting a physician. All matters of health require medical supervision, Neither the author nor the publisher shall be liable or responsible for any loss or damage allegedly arising from any information or suggestions in this book.

Neither the publisher nor the author is responsible for specific health or allergy needs that may require medical supervision or for any adverse reaction to the recipes herein. While the author has made every effort to provide accurate internet addresses at the time of publication, neither the publisher nor the author assumes any responsibility for errors, or for changes that occur after publication. Further, neither the publisher nor author assumes any responsibility for third-party websites or their content.

ENDORSEMENTS

"CONQUER THYSELF is an inspiring story of beating terminal cancer and a practical guide to staying healthy, complete with nutrition and exercise tips. Researchers have proven that food choices can help prevent cancer and, when cancer has been diagnosed, nutrition can improve survival. This book will show you just how easy it is to live a healthful life."

Neal D. Barnard, MD
President, Physicians Committee for Responsible Medicine
Adjunct Associate Professor of Medicine
George Washington University

"D. A. Metrov shares his unique insights as well as the practical steps he took to stop terminal cancer in its tracks, banish it from his body, and restore himself to remarkable health and wellness. *Conquer Thyself* is an inspirational story that marches on the front lines of America's growing Health Revolution."

John Westerdahl, Ph.D., M.P.H., R.D., C.N.S.
Director, Bragg Health Institute
Radio Talk Show Host, Health & Longevity

"CONQUER THYSELF is the key to becoming whole. Mr. Metrov shares his journey of recovery from cancer with simple straight-forward guidelines; yet deeply profound. Readers can benefit from his exemplary lifestyle."

Benjamin Lau, MD, PhD
Emeritus Professor, Loma Linda University

"I thought I was leading a healthy lifestyle. Then I contracted one of the worst cancers known to man. I'm now cancer-free. I developed heart problems as a result of prescription cancer and pain medications. I was able to reverse my heart disease without surgery, stents, or additional medications. This book contains the system I used to regain and maintain my health. If it worked for me, it can work for you." ~ *D. A. Metrov*

- Are you fed up with going to the doctor's and taking medications?

- Have you had it with being in the hospital?

- Are you willing to do anything to regain your health?

- Are you fed up with paying medical bills?

- Are you obese or overweight, and have no idea why?

- Are you appalled by your weight, but have no idea what to do about it?

- Would you like to be a model of good health instead of plagued by sickness and disease?

- Would you like to be part of the solution to the world's health care dilemma rather than part of the problem?

- Would you like to be able to run, and jump, and shout for joy like you did when you were a kid?

- Would you like to be of service to your fellow man instead of a burden to your family and society?

YOU CAN GET WELL!

CONTENTS

OVERALL SUMMARY

Medical science is learning that many, if not most, common diseases are a result of our eating and lifestyle habits. Welcome to the basics of *Health by Design*.

In this book I'll explore the hypothesis that good health is determined by a synergy of three fundamental factors: Proper Diet, Exercise, and Stress (or mind) Management.

By ingesting a nutrient-dense, non-toxic diet, my body will look, feel, and function at its best which will in turn affect my mental outlook in a positive way.

By exercising regularly, my body will maintain strength, balance, and optimal circulation which will also improve my body's functionality and my mental outlook.

By keeping stress (fear) in check, my mind will enjoy greater joy and serenity sending positive messages to my body which will in turn maximize my immune system's ability to destroy disease.

Mind and body work hand-in-hand to achieve ultimate efficiency... or self-annihilation.

"Conquer thyself, till thou has done this, thou art but a slave."
~ Sir Richard Francis Burton, British Explorer, 1821-1890

FOREWORD

At the age of 61, I was diagnosed with one of the deadliest, most aggressive prostate cancers known to man. I could provide its scientific name, but I'd rather not give it another nit of attention. After receiving the news from my urologist, I Googled this particular malady, and discovered that only eight men in the history of medicine had ever had it before me. They were all dead within weeks of being diagnosed. I figured I was a goner.

Two days later, I was walking alone through the woods pondering the ostensibly short remainder of my earthly existence. I was weary of my life-long struggle to succeed as an artist, and surprisingly unafraid of dying. I was ready to "throw in the towel." Without warning, I heard a voice in my head: "You don't think I'm going to let you die, do you?"

I'm not accustomed to hearing voices in my head, and this one was particularly clear. I had no idea who the voice belonged to, though I suspected (and still do) it was the voice of my personal Higher Power. The moment I heard it, I knew I was going to be okay. On that same walk, I had the crystal clear realization that, on the deepest level of my being, the choice to live or die was mine. I decided to kick cancer's ass.

I had to undergo a series of "cures." Because of the rarity of this cancer, my oncology team wasn't quite sure what to do with me. They decided to bombard me with as much chemo and radiation as possible just short of killing me. Not to downplay the importance of these treatments in saving my life, I was surprised to discover the techniques of "modern" medicine had not much improved over the practice of Medieval Blood Letting. At least that's how it seemed. (One "specialist" wanted to carve out half my innards, including my anus, as a final precaution. I respectfully declined.) Chemo and radiation are methods of killing cancer cells. But they also kill and damage an inordinate number of healthy cells while they're at it. It's a nasty business that you want to avoid if you can.

Most people never fully recover from such high-tech punishment. However, today, I'm probably more full of life and vigor than ever before. And that's why I decided to write this book. I not only want to share what I've learned, I also wanted a simple, concise way to remind myself of the few things I need to do in order to stay healthy, fit, and most importantly, in a state of inner peace... or at least as much as possible.

I'm not a certified doctor or nutritionist. I'm simply a man who's learned a great deal about certain things (often the "hard way") because of my passionate and determined nature. I'm writing this book to share my experiences and to document what has worked for me. I do not prescribe treatments or cures, so please don't write me asking for any. You should consult a medical doctor if you are experiencing any prolonged ailments.

Throughout this small book, you'll come across the word, "discipline," and hence derives the title: CONQUER THYSELF. I have come to believe that in order to learn, grow, and maintain maximum efficiency, we need to work at it. Since we are essentially comfort-seeking creatures, work takes effort and desire. The problem is, most of us, including myself, won't do the work (that is change our lifestyles), unless faced with a serious, life-threatening health crisis. Hopefully, this book will help convince you not to wait that long. Or if you've already experienced the crisis, I hope the words that follow—the lessons I've learned and the practices I maintain— may help you avoid another. If they end up working for you, then make them your own.

CHAPTER ONE
DIET

"What you eat and drink today, is walking and talking tomorrow."
~ From the Bragg Healthy Lifestyle

When I was diagnosed with terminal cancer, I was working as webmaster and videographer for Bragg Live Food Products in Santa Barbara, California. Founded by Dr. Paul C. Bragg in 1912, Bragg claims to be the oldest "health" company in America. I was comfortable at Bragg. I'd always been conscious about eating well and staying fit. I always tried to exercise daily. I'd been a wrestling champion in high school, and had won an athletic scholarship to UCLA. No one in my family had ever had cancer. To say the diagnosis was a shock is an understatement..

About fifteen years earlier I'd begun to practice the "Zone Diet" which prescribes that 75% of one's diet should be protein. It also suggested that chicken breast was the best source of protein. Not long ago, the Physicians Committee for Responsible Medicine (www.pcrm.org) announced that grilled chicken causes cancer. This brave, pioneer group of conscious doctors even filed a law suit against fast food companies that sell grilled chicken. Of course, I wondered if my strict adherence to the Zone Diet had been instrumental in giving me cancer.

Additionally, we know today that too much animal protein can cause cancer. And if we're talking about commercially raised chicken (or any livestock), we must consider the effects of antibiotics, pesticides, GMOs, growth hormones, even the arsenic used to kill parasites and give chicken flesh a more appealing color.

Carcinogens seem to be everywhere in our environment these days—in our water, food, atmosphere, the earth, even in the very airwaves.

In reference to my struggles to "succeed as an artist" mentioned in the foreword, I had lived in a state of chronic stress for over twenty-five years due to my determination to "make it" in the movie business. I'll discuss stress more in Chapter Three as I believe this plays an even more important role in health than diet and nutrition.

Still, I believe that working at Bragg saved my life. Under the supervision of Dr. John Westerdahl, Bragg's Director of Health Science, it was part of my daily responsibilities to post the latest nutrition reports on the Bragg website. (www.bragg.com).

Dr. Westerdahl has committed his life to staying abreast of the latest developments in health and nutrition. He became my nutrition guru and mentor. Before, during, and after my cancer treatment, I was able to pick his brain on the subject. He is a veritable walking encyclopedia of information.

So I learned from articles by experts, reports by scientists and scientific study groups; from discussions with Dr. Westerdahl, and from seminal books like "The China Study" by Dr. T. Colin Campbell, "Prevent and Reverse Heart Disease" by Dr. Caldwell B. Esselstyn Jr., and "The Spectrum," by Dr. Dean Ornish. I became determined to beat my cancer, and also to ensure that it would never return. I am confident it will not.

I devoured all the information I could find. I like to believe I know more than the average doctor about preventative medicine. I say this only because the doctors I've observed have barely enough time to read their respective medical journals, let alone study non-AMA approved literature on alternative practices and break-through nutrition discoveries.

And perhaps worse, it would appear that either directly or indirectly, the "medical" journals are published by Big Pharma, the major pharmaceutical companies which also, by the way, financed the building of most of the medical schools in this country. Of course, it is decidedly NOT in the interests of these mega-corporations to inform people they can stay healthy by simple lifestyle choices. These corporations don't make money from personal lifestyle choices, they make money by selling prescription medications and high-technology. Much could be written about the questionable practices now taking place in this country that filter down from Big Pharma, through the FDA, the American Medical Association, hospitals, and countless cancer, diabetes, heart, and other "health" related organizations. Because of the influence of Big Business, we can no longer count on the FDA to protect or guarantee the safety of our food. We're on our own, folks.

Further discussion of Big Business, however, is beyond the scope of this book. Let it suffice to say that a large number of revealing documentaries on these subjects can be found on Netflix. "Food, Inc," and "The Corporation," are a couple to get you started.

Since my experience was with cancer, you may ask why I mention a book on heart disease. The answer is, I had to take pain medications for the year during and following my cancer treatment. Yes, the process was unduly painful. Yet because of the pain medication I was able to continue working and exercising daily.

When it came time to wean off the pain meds, I discovered to my dismay that I was suddenly experiencing angina from the least bit of exertion. Angina is a painful constriction in the chest area brought about by insufficient blood flow through the heart arteries. At times it was so bad, it brought me to my knees in agony. It felt like I was having a full blown heart attack. What's this? I thought. I've always been in good shape. Always tried to eat well and exercise daily. How can I be having heart problems?

When I visited a cardiologist, he said two of my main heart arteries were partially blocked. He recommended immediate quadruple bypass surgery. I told him I'd think about it. I came to believe that somehow the pain medication, or I should say, withdrawing from the pain medication, left me with inflamed arteries, thus restricting my blood flow. *(Update: I've since discovered chemo and radiation can also cause "long term" adverse affects on one's heart, i.e. side effects that don't appear until 7-8 years later. Happy to report, these have also been resolved using the principles in this book.)* When I mentioned the problem to Dr. Westerdahl, he said to me, without hesitation, "You may have to stop using olive oil."

"Huh? Olive oil is supposed to be good for your heart." Dr. Westerdahl went on to describe several heart disease reversal programs that take people off all oils. Apparently, olive oil is not so "good" for your heart as the "Greek Diet" advocates would lead you to believe. It's simply not as bad as some of the other oils available on the market. The Greeks suffer from as many heart attacks as most other Westerners.

Sure enough, I stopped olive oil, and immediately the angina attacks subsided dramatically.

Besides quitting oils, I knew there were other alternatives to heart surgery. I knew I had to change my diet. I knew Dr. Esselstyn and Dr. Dean Ornish had been successful in reversing heart disease by putting their patients on plant-based or Vegan diets, which means no animal foods including red meat, chicken, fish, cheese, and dairy. President Bill Clinton is probably the most famous example of a man who reversed his heart disease by switching to a plant-based diet. (Ten years after proving he could reverse heart disease with a plant-based diet, Dean Ornish further proved he could reverse certain cancers the same way.)

Today, I consider myself a Vegan. Not only do I feel great, but I've lost weight and have more energy. When I made the commitment to eating a plant-based diet, I discovered that my lifelong mentor, Leonardo da Vinci, ate the same way. Apparently, so did Benjamin Franklin and Einstein. Good role models, eh?

"Nothing will benefit human health and increase the chances for survival of life on earth as much as the evolution to a vegetarian diet."
~ Albert Einstein

I also admire the Hunzas whose diet consists entirely of fruits, vegetables, grains, and small portions of meat, but only on special occasions, about once a month. In case you haven't heard of the Hunzas, they are a simple people who live high in the Himalayas, in the so-called Lost Valley of Shangri-La. They typically live to be centenarians, some even living to 120, continuing to perform rigorous physical labor almost to the end.

Sometimes people tell me they wouldn't want to live to 120. I agree. No one would want to live that long unless they were feeling pretty good and having a pretty darn good time. Perhaps such a life is only possible in a remote, paradisiacal valley cut off from the stresses of modern day life. Or maybe, with some practice and effort, it might be possible anywhere.

I highly recommend Dr. Campbell's book, "The China Study." To summarize, Dr. Campbell spent forty years researching nutrition. After rigorous study and countless tests, he concluded that animal proteins nurture cancer, while plants, i.e. fruits and vegetables, contain attributes that can kill and prevent cancer (as well as a plethora of other diseases which most Americans now consider simply a part of life, such as diabetes, strokes, heart disease, obesity, Parkinson's, and so on. These diseases are NOT simply part of life. They are typically brought about by lifestyle choices, specifically eating habits, many of which have been sold to us as being "healthy.") Dr. Campbell further demonstrated that in order to "starve," or prevent cancer, animal protein must not exceed 5% of our overall diet. In his lectures, I understand he advocates a completely animal-free diet. Unfortunately, Americans have been brainwashed to eat far too much animal protein. Because of powerful cattle, poultry, and dairy lobbyists, the U.S. Government (i.e. we taxpayers) subsidizes those industries. That's why a sirloin steak is now cheaper than a head of organic broccoli.

There is a revolution underway that is changing our understanding of how to be healthy. It's being brought about by those seeking to explain the epidemic of disease that's ravaging the United States today. How is it that the most "modern" society on the planet has an average life span of only seventy-eight years old? Something is wrong with this picture.

The bottom line is this: now, nearly four years following my cancer treatment, I am cancer-free, strong, radiant, and healthy. I no longer suffer angina even though I exercise daily with the vigor of a collegiate athlete. (Okay, I exaggerate slightly, but I'm in pretty darn good shape.) It's not only because of my physical lifestyle, but also because of my mental and spiritual practices which I will discuss in subsequent chapters.

The following list contains the plant-based foods I've decided are healthiest for me. And I say, "healthiest for me," because I've come to believe that not one size fits all. In other words, everyone's physical make-up is slightly different. For example, some people may have a bad reaction to certain grains, others to certain vegetables. Each of us must make the effort to determine what works best for us. There are endless resources online where you can look up the nutritional value of any food. I'm sure you can find many to add to my list. The one thing I would strongly suggest is that whatever you eat, make sure it's certified organic.

MOST IMPORTANT VEGETABLES

Cabbage
Collard Greens
Onion
Garlic (possibly the King of Cancer Killers)
Spinach
Broccoli (cancer killer)
Cauliflower
Carrots (cancer killer)
Peas
Kale
Beans
Cucumber
Sweet Potato
Swiss Chard
Tomato
Zucchini
Brussels Sprouts
Egg Plant
Asparagus (cancer killer)
Brown Rice
Mushrooms

Bok Choy
Sea Vegetables (for trace minerals not found anywhere else)

MOST IMPORTANT FRUITS

Strawberries
Blueberries
Raisins
Apples
Oranges
Grapefruit
Grapes
Bananas
Mango
Watermelon
Apricots
Cantaloupe
Cherries
Goji Berries
Acai Berries
Peach
Pear
Pomegranate
Cranberries (cancer killer)
Lemons

IMPORTANT SUPPLEMENTS

Multi-vitamin & minerals
Vitamin D
Vitamin E
Vitamin C
Beta Sitosterol (to reduce cholesterol)
Ginseng
Magnesium
Potassium

Iodine (from Salmon)
(Note: Many researchers now believe a diet rich in fruits and vegetables will provide all the vitamins & minerals we need; in fact these nutrients are most beneficial when ingested as whole foods.)

OTHER

Whole Grains
Walnuts
Wheat germ
Barley
Spirulina
Wheat Grass (cancer killer)
Nutritional Yeast (B12)
Cinnamon
Nuts
Cayenne pepper (Vitamin A; reduces inflammation)
Stevia (my sweetener of choice)
Raw, Organic Honey
Organic Apple Cider Vinegar

A note about apple cider vinegar: This remarkable elixir was used by Hippocrates, the Father of Medicine, to cure almost everything imaginable. As Bragg webmaster, I received endless *unsolicited* testimonials from people the world over reporting that ACV had resolved their health issues—internal & external—where modern medicines had failed. (See the "Testimonials" section on www.bragg.com.) Yet, there is little scientific evidence as to why ACV is so potent except that it raises the body's alkalinity level. We know diseases thrive in acidic environments. (We also know that animal foods elevate the body's acidity, whereas vegetables raise alkalinity—another argument for the Vegan diet). Perhaps once the body reduces acidity and achieves a higher alkaline state, the immune system is simply better empowered to banish disease.

The above food list is by no means exhaustive. In fact, I'm constantly revising it for my own personal use. Use it as a place to start your healthy lifestyle. Go easy on the salt. Keep sugar, fat, and animal protein (meat, chicken, fish, dairy, eggs) to 5% or less of your overall diet if you consume it at all. And make sure all foods are ORGANIC. Another part of my education has been to learn that most commercials foods are no longer healthy, and many are simply unfit for human consumption.

If you're eating this way for the first time, it will probably take some discipline for you to stay on the straight and narrow. The big food corporations (and there are now only a handful controlling the world's food supply) have discovered how to make food addictive, and hence to sell more of it. The fats, salts, and sugars (not to mention the chemicals, pesticides, GMOs, MSG, and growth hormones) are like powerful drugs. We've all been hooked, and it'll take work to break the habits.

It was my own personal experience that once I stopped daily consumption of animal products, I really began to TASTE for the first time in my life. I came to enjoy the flavor of vegetables, raw or steamed. Before I became totally Vegan, I began to dislike how animal foods made me feel. I realized they slowed me down and made me feel clogged up, is the best way to describe it. The last thing I want to be is "clogged up." Eastern medicine teaches that all physical disorders are due to some blockage in circulation or "flow." Whether it be the flow of blood, fluids, digestive processes, oxygen, or Chi, circulation must not be restricted, otherwise the system grows ill or dis-eased.

Look at the Universe—from the smallest sub-nuclear particles to the blood in our veins, to the myriad stars in the sky—everything is moving in an endless, circular, and harmonious flow.

I prefer to eat three meals a day with maybe a small, healthy snack or two, such as nuts or dried fruit, in between. While in my experience it's possible to gain weight even on a plant-based diet, it's not easy, so I'm not overly concerned about portions. The "Forks Over Knives" newsletter (www.forksoverknives.com) regularly publishes before and after photos of people who were once obese and who switched to a plant-based diet losing hundreds of pounds.

Of course there are a wide variety of diets and theories out there about the healthiest ways to eat, including eating more protein, less protein, more carbs, less carbs, more fat, less fat, more meat, less meat, no meat, etc, etc. I'm not interested in debating any of this. Once again, I'm sharing what works for me personally. I suggest you do the same—find out what works for you.

Considering all the different, possible physiological make-ups of the human body, all the different foods, organic vs non-organic, all the different *combinations* of foods, *quantities* of foods, plus environmental and genetic factors, the Science of Nutrition is very complex indeed. I haven't found anyone who's completely mastered it yet, and I doubt anyone ever will. Perhaps someday a highly sophisticated computer program may come close, but that is still a ways off.

I've become wary of diet and nutrition fads. I've seen the most acclaimed diets debunked, and almost every trend come and go. According to my research, the only "weight-loss diet" that really works is one that entails keeping a small notebook, writing down everything that's eaten during the course of a day, and tallying up the calories. This may be effective for losing weight, but, if the *quality* of food is not taken into consideration, this approach may not necessarily be the healthiest.

Lastly, keep plenty of fluids in your body. Get into the habit of drinking several glasses of water every day. The first thing I do in the morning is drink a full, eight-ounce glass of water. Again, get into the habit, because as you get older, you may start to forget. I can't tell you how many elderly people I've known who forget to drink water. They feel awful, and don't know why. Their doctor will often prescribe some ridiculous medication, when all they need to do is hydrate.

Actually, the best way to keep fluids in your system is by eating fruits and other plant-based foods. Water, by itself, tends to go through you rather quickly. The water in fruits and vegetables stays in your system longer, and hence our body has more time to extract and utilize it.

Fluids are part of maintaining good circulation. Think about a drain pipe that's all mucked up with little washing through it. It's not going to drain too well, is it? By the way—on the subject of draining—by by eating a plant-based diet, keeping fluids in your system and exercising regularly, you're not likely to have any elimination problems.

Stay hydrated. You won't always want to drink water, but make yourself do it. Practice discipline. Conquer Yourself. Put up signs in your kitchen if you have to: DRINK! Not only will you feel better, you'll look better because your skin cells need water to stay young and healthy.

And while we're on the subject of fluids, I don't drink alcohol (or do drugs). It's pretty well established that alcohol fuels some diseases like cancer, in particular. Most oncologists these days will recommend that their patients give up alcohol for a better chance of recovery. Alcohol is also known to kill brain cells.

VEGANISM AND THE ENVIRONMENT

Veganism, or eating a plant-based diet, is good for the environment for numerous reasons. It's been estimated that livestock contribute 18% of all greenhouse gas emissions. They are also responsible for 64% of the ammonia emissions that contribute to acid rain. Commercial livestock has been identified as the largest sectoral source of water pollution, not only from manure, but from antibiotics and hormones, chemicals from tanneries, fertilizers and pesticides used for feed crops, and tainted sediments from eroded pastures. Much of the world's deforestation is taking place to create more grazing area for livestock. The filthy, cruel conditions under which livestock—cattle, chickens, pigs—are penned and slaughtered, is reason enough to stop eating commercially raised animals.

MEALS

My intention is not to write a recipe book, there are already plenty out there, a few of which I'll list in the back of the book. I just want to share some of my personal eating habits.

BREAKFAST

I love making a super cereal bowl for breakfast. I chop up and add the following:

- (1) Apple ("An apple a day keeps the doctor away." There's a reason this saying has been around so long... apples are an excellent source of nutrients. But apples tend to soak up and retain pesticides, so only eat organic varieties.)

- ½ Banana

- (1) Tablespoon Organic Wheat Germ (Eliminate this if you have gluten intolerance, which is actually rare, by the way, but has become quite the rage lately.)

- (1) Teaspoon Ground Organic Flaxseed

- (1) Teaspoon Turmeric (reduces inflammation.)

- (1) Tablespoon Cinnamon (improves memory)

- (3) Walnuts (According to legend, Daniel Boone raved about walnuts, claiming they alone kept him marching through the wilderness for weeks at a time.)

- ½ Cup Oat Bran (excellent for keeping your LDL—known as "bad" cholesterol—low)

- ½ Cup whole grain cereal of your choice

• (2) Tablespoons of Raisins or Blueberries (Excellent source of antioxidants)

• Organic Stevia (To taste; make sure it's not cut with casein or other dairy powder.)

• (1) Teaspoon Organic Cocoa Powder (Optional—will require more sweetening)

• Any Kind of Berries (Optional)

Add water and/or organic soy milk.

Because I get up very early to write, I usually have several cups of green tea with almond milk before breakfast—green tea being another potent cancer killer. There seems to be an on-going debate on the healthiness of coffee. I will sometimes have a cup during the day, but not too often.

LUNCH

I almost always have a tossed, green salad for lunch. Some of my usual ingredients include:

• Mixed Green Leafs (Usually Arugula and Kale.)

• Tomatoes

• Onions (I prefer the red variety.)

• Carrots (Known to be potent cancer killers, I try to eat at least one or two a day.)

• ½ Avocado (These add great flavor to your salad, but go easy on them, they are fatty. And yes, even the "good" fat can add to your waistline.)

Since I'm on an oil-free diet, I use non-fat dressings on my salad. I love Bragg's "Braggberry" or "Hawaiian" non-fat, oil-free dressings, but I add a few squirts of Bragg Coconut Aminos for the extra flavor. And you can certainly add or change-up the ingredients. Just about any veggie that can be eaten raw can be mixed into a salad, as well as nuts and fruits like apple slices and raisins.

Some people tire of eating the same thing every day, but I always enjoy a healthy salad. If you like to mix things up, see the Suggested Reading section in the back of the book for other recipe options.

DINNER

For some reason dinner is usually the meal I prefer to change once in awhile, though, because of my schedule, I usually make a big pot of something—several days worth—keep it in a large container in the fridge, and microwave my evening portion. Some of my favorite dishes are:

STEAMED VEGETABLES. Like salads, you can mix and combine just about anything that will steam to edible consistency in 5-10 minutes. I love broccoli (another potent cancer killer), potatoes (all different colors), cabbage, onions, garlic, asparagus, zucchini, mushrooms, and bell peppers (all colors).
After steaming, I toss them and season with Bragg Coconut Aminos and Bragg Nutritional Yeast which seem to add plenty of flavor.

STEAMED VEGETABLES/RICE. Spoon the above veggies over organic, brown rice. I love to mix brown and wild rice, then make sure to add minced, fresh garlic.

RICE & BEANS/FRESH SALSA. A simple, but healthy (and filling) meal. Garnish with your favorite flavors.

WHOLE GRAIN PASTA. Again, if you have gluten or wheat allergies, you'll want to avoid this one, but there are substitutes like rice pasta. Of course, there are countless toppings for pasta, one of my favorites being sautéed tomatoes and garlic. You can even top your pasta with plain, steamed vegetables for a very tasty meal.

As you may have guessed by now, I've come to love eating simply. Besides, I don't have much patience for cooking. I enjoy good taste, but the nutritional quality of my food trumps everything else. Again, if you like to spend time in the kitchen, I have some awesome cookbooks in the "Suggested Reading" section.

Am I a purist, sticking to my Vegan diet 100% of the time, day in and day out? For the most part, yes. Let's put it this way... I do my best. Don't beat yourself up if you slip now and then. Just get back in the saddle, and keep on riding.

DESSERT

My favorite dessert is to simply mix up a bowl of chopped strawberries, add raisins, and sweeten with a little Stevia. Of course you can do the same thing with any combination of berries. And you can add some almond milk if you like.

DRINK

I mostly drink good old water. It should be pure spring water, distilled, or filtered through a reverse osmosis system to make sure it's not fluoridated or otherwise contaminated with pollutants. I also make a lemonade from 2-3 fresh, squeezed lemons, 4 oz. apple cider vinegar, cayenne pepper, and honey. I make a two-quart pitcher at a time, combining these ingredients to my taste, and keep it in the fridge.

A note about Stevia: For most people (me included), Stevia is an acquired taste, especially if you're a reformed sugar-lover. However, after a lot of experimentation, I've discovered the secret of using Stevia is to use just the right amount for various dishes. It's VERY strong stuff and can be up to 300 times sweeter than sugar! But according to my research, it's really the only healthy, zero-calorie, sugar-free sweetener to use. It's natural and comes from plant leaves. I can't tell you how happy I am to be almost completely OFF sugar.

A note about sugar and salt: Make sure to use these in moderation. I've observed on the rare occasions I've inadvertently used too much sugar or salt (or oil, which is often hard to avoid, especially if you eat out), I've felt a tinge of angina if I exercise afterwards. I've always read that salt and sugar are not good for heart health, but it's surprising how quickly their adverse effects can be felt.

A note on eating out: I've learned most restaurants will steam your vegetables for you instead of cooking them with oils.

A note about chocolate: Doesn't everyone LOVE chocolate? Okay, it has one of the highest antioxidant levels of any food, but it's also very high in fat and sugar. Pure cocoa powder rocks in terms of its nutritional value, but it's very bitter. I only eat chocolate on very rare occasions.

THE PROBLEM WITH JUNK FOOD

So-called "Junk Food" contains ingredients that make us want to eat more of it! It contains ingredients that can get us hooked! Ingredients that are addictive! Fat, salt, sugar, and MSG are addictive and damaging to our bodies. High fructose corn syrup is not only in junk food, but in almost ALL PROCESSED FOODS. It has been linked to weight gain, obesity, type 2 diabetes, metabolic syndrome, high triglyceride levels, hardening of the arteries, and heart disease. Some medical experts consider it the biggest contributor to disease in the world today. If you're hooked on junk food, you need to get off it. It may not be easy. It will take determination and effort. You may even have to join a support group like Overeaters Anonymous. Google this to find groups near you.

We are stubborn... especially about the food we eat. We don't want advice about our eating habits. Again, most of us won't change until we're hit with a major health crisis, like being diagnosed with a serious, life-threatening disease. Unfortunately, if you're reading this book, chances are you're probably already sick.

CHAPTER SUMMARY

My research has led me to believe that an organic, plant-based diet is the healthiest and most nutritious way for me to eat.

CHAPTER TWO
EXERCISE

"Most people work at dying. I work at living. It's a pain in the ass. You have to eat right and exercise."
~ Jack LaLanne

I can already tell this is going to be a short chapter. It simply comes down to this: Move! A lot! (By the way, if you don't know who Jack LaLanne is, he's the guy who invented the gymnasium and the workout machine. Before him, there was no such thing as "working out." He opened the first gym in America in 1936. He went on to host his own television fitness show that aired for almost 35 years. He credited Paul C. Bragg for launching his lifelong passion for health and wellness. Jack LaLanne is nothing less than the Father of Modern Day Fitness. We love you, Jack!)

Do you know that your body is approximately 60% water? What happens to water that doesn't keep moving? It becomes stagnant. The dictionary defines *stagnant* as "... stale or foul from standing; inactive, sluggish, or dull." Stagnant water is the best breeding ground for bacteria and parasites.

To a certain extent, we all have inertia. Because of a mysterious thing called gravity, it takes effort to get up and move. But if we don't do it, like any body of water, we tend to stagnate. Our physiological commerce comes to a halt. Our systems go bust.

I was a wrestling champion in high school. Before that, I had no interest in sports. My father was not a sports enthusiast so we never watched sporting events like football or baseball in my house. I was a skinny, uncoordinated sophomore at Chaffey High in Ontario, California when the school wrestling coach approached me. For some reason, he thought I'd make a good wrestler. He invited me to try out for the team. I did and liked it.

That summer, when school was out (I was 15), I got a job working for the Italian brick mason who lived across the street. He used to drop me off at the job site where, for example, he was contracted to build an eight bay, auto repair shop. A large transport truck would drop off pallets containing tens of thousands of cinder blocks. The mason would explain to me it was my job to move the cinder blocks (two at a time, one in each hand), to strategic positions up on the scaffolding which rose three levels off the ground all around the building site. He would then jump in his truck and drive off. I wouldn't see him again until he returned at the end of the day to pick me up.

The summer heat was sweltering, as Ontario sits on the edge of the Mojave desert. Being a dutiful lad, I positioned the cinder blocks, two at a time, day after day, until they were all in their proper places. This meant that when the mason went to work, all he had to do was spread a trowel-full of cement with one hand and plop a cinder block in its slot with the other. And if he had to reach too far, I was in trouble! While he did that, the next phase of my job was to make sure his "mud" or concrete was sitting on the mixing board next to him, and remained the proper consistency at all times. In other words, my duty was to make sure that he exerted himself as little as possible.

This routine was repeated for cinder block walls, fireplaces, chimneys, and other types of structures all summer long. When wrestling season began the following year, I quickly made the varsity team. Not only did my strength far surpass that of the average male athlete, I was born quick with a natural sense of balance. My opponents never had a chance.

There's another reason I was a champion wrestler. My father was "old school." He was a first generation American who'd grown up on the mean streets of Chicago in the 1930's. I loved the man, but I could never earn his approval. Growing up, all I heard from him was how worthless I was. In short, by today's standards, he was psychologically and physically abusive. The result was, despite the fact I was a meek, well-behaved kid, I developed a mean streak by the time I reached my teen years. So between my physical attributes and said meanness, I was, to say the least, formidable on the mat.

But no matter how many medals I won, my father never let on that he was proud of me. I never won that pat on the back I so desperately craved. I carried doubts about my self-worth into adulthood. This would become one of the major reasons I eventually contracted cancer which I will address in detail in the chapter on stress management. I should mention I've done a lot of work to forgive my father, doing so repeatedly over the years.

Back to exercise: I always had a natural inclination to eat healthy and stay physically fit. As already mentioned, this alone was not enough to prevent a life-threatening disease, but these are crucial elements to good health.

Exercising not only pumps oxygen—the Invisible Staff of Life—to our cells, but also forces our oxygen-carrying blood to flow to more places in greater quantities, hence improving circulation, nurturing, and cleansing waste from the body. There are far more benefits from exercise, more scientific in nature, that I could research and list here. But for me, it's enough to know that exercise aids Good Circulation which aids Good Health. Oh, yes, and it helps reduce stress.

I know of two main types of exercise: Aerobic and anaerobic. Basically aerobic exercise means you elevate your heart and respiratory rate for at least twenty minutes in order to achieve its benefits which, according to the Mayo Clinic, are:

- Keeps excess pounds at bay
- Increases your stamina
- Wards off viral illnesses
- Reduces your health risks
- Manages chronic conditions
- Strengthens your heart
- Keeps your arteries clear
- Boosts your mood
- Keeps you active and independent as you age
- Live longer

All these benefits are brought about by increased blood circulation and oxygen in the body. If you're not doing daily aerobic exercise now, start slowly and work your way up to at least twenty minutes a day. I've listened to interviews with very fit 90+ year olds who walk at least three miles a day. My wife and I used to hike in the Eastern Sierra mountains, and be embarrassed by smiling couples in their 80's who passed us going UP the mountain. I've also known people this same age who never exercised at all and can barely move even using a walker. The lesson: Use It Or Lose It.

My best understanding is that anaerobic exercise takes place when we're putting stress on our muscles for short bursts of time, like weight training. These bursts of muscle stress are good for building muscle and hence body strength, but don't have all the benefits of aerobic exercise.

I try to exercise daily for at least 30-60 minutes. If ever I'm feeling a little run down or too sore, I may take off a day here and there to let my body rest. I practiced Tae Bo for years. I loved it. But it involves a lot of jumping up and down, which in my case, caused one of my spinal discs to collapse. Not good. The collapsed disc impinged on a nerve which not only caused pain but numbness in one leg. Okay... no more jumping up and down for this camper. I love to ride my mountain bike. It's far less impact on my joints. But after years of doing so, I started to feel I was getting plenty of lower body exercise, but not enough upper body. As of this writing, I now try to swim several days a week, as well as bike-ride. Oh, and 50 pushups every morning.

Swimming employs more muscles, upper and lower, and is probably the least strain on joints. It's a great aerobic exercise which means I'm getting lots of blood and oxygen pumped through my system. Plus I sweat even though I'm in the water which is good for purging toxins.

I suspect that exercising 30-60 minutes a day is not really enough. Remember the Hunzas who perform physical labor almost daily their entire lives? In my world, I spend most of my time sitting at a computer. I need to force myself to get up and move around more.

I've discovered the importance of s-t-r-e-t-c-h-i-n-g, especially as I get older. I need to remember to stretch because otherwise I tend to stiffen up. Stiff is not good. Stay limber. Every morning, while waiting for my tea water to boil, I do a quick, mini-yoga session in the kitchen. Every morning! After drinking a full glass of water, I bend over and touch my toes. I circle my arms backward and forward. I slowly swivel my skull around on my neck. Shake out my hands. Twist my torso back and forth (good for balance, by the way). I squat to stretch out my groin. Don't tell my wife, but I put the backs of my heels, one by one, up on the counter and push my head down toward my knee, stretching out my hamstrings, knee joint, and lower back. I squat down and push back one leg at a time, again stretching out my groin. I would benefit greatly from a full on yoga session daily, but face it, who has time for aerobic exercise and yoga every day?

Establish a routine for yourself—a daily routine if possible. Even when you're not exercising, remember to breathe deeply often. I doubt you can get too much oxygen into your blood by normal means. But get in an official exercise session at least once a day. You won't always feel like doing it. Like Jack LaLanne used to say, "It's a pain in the ass." But make yourself. Practice discipline and it will pay off. Good old Jack worked out to the end and he was in pretty damned good shape until he left us at age 96.

EXERCISES

SWIMMING

As already mentioned, I prefer swimming above all other exercises because its aerobic, works the most muscles and organs, upper and lower, and has the least harmful impact on my body.

BIKE RIDING

I prefer to ride my mountain bike off road, on dirt trails, otherwise, I'm breathing in too much car exhaust. I also like my bike because there's little jarring of my spine and joints.

JOGGING

I'm not a big fan of jogging, especially as I get older. But I've always felt it's better to jog on grass or dirt, otherwise the impact from running on asphalt or concrete can be harmful to your spine and knee joints.

WALKING

I believe Power-Walking is probably just as beneficial as jogging. I like to stretch my arms up and down as I walk to get in some upper body work. Warning: Don't do this when there are people approaching you in the distance. They'll think you're waving for help and it will cause unnecessary alarm and confusion!

HIKING

My wife and I love hiking. As opposed to simply walking on a level surface, hiking usually includes uphill and downhill. Besides, I enjoy the sights of Nature which are a constant source of serenity, fascination, and beauty.

WEIGHT LIFTING

For me, weight lifting was more important when I was younger and wanting to build strength. I don't do it that much anymore, though it probably wouldn't hurt in moderation. I just feel I get more benefit from aerobic, oxygen-infusing, exercise.

WRESTLING

I still love to wrestle... in my dreams. I always imagine I can still wrestle just about anyone on the planet. Thankfully, I have enough sense not to. I would probably hurt myself. Sigh, I do miss it.

AKIDO

I studied Akido for awhile, and loved it. It's my favorite martial art in terms of its philosophy which is based on non-resistance. I always think about getting back into it.

TAI CHI

I do Tai Chi once in awhile. It's a gentle work out, and requires patience. Most of the moves are performed slowly. Normally, I enjoy something a little more rigorous.

YOGA

Yoga rocks. You can go fast or slow as long as you're thorough. I've come to understand that as I age, stretching grows in importance, otherwise, I seem to get stiffer by the day! Stiff is not good. Limber is good. I need to stretch. Also, there are apparently spiritual benefits from practicing yoga, but for me, those are hard to define. The simplest yoga move is bending over and touching your toes. I do it often.

OTHER EXERCISES

Naturally, there are countless ways to exercise. There are group exercises and individual exercises. Do your homework and find out what works best for you. If you don't know where to start, you can join your local gym. Besides weight lifting and aerobic machines, they usually offer a variety of classes and even personal training programs.

CHAPTER SUMMARY

I want my body to stay strong and fit. Besides strength, I need fresh oxygen and proper circulation for optimal health. The best way to achieve this is through exercise.

CHAPTER THREE
STRESS MANAGEMENT

"He who conquers a thousand men a thousand times is nothing compared to he who conquers himself."
~ Siddharta Gautama

WHAT IS REALITY?

Like many of us, I was deeply intrigued by the movie, "The Secret." Its message: We should visualize what we want, and practice feeling like we already have it in order to manifest our dreams. The reason I responded to this message was because I'd been familiar with it my entire life.

Early on, I was introduced to "The Power of Positive Thinking" by Norman Vincent Peale. Its message is evident in the title. As a boy, even as an adult, I never fully grasped this message for a very long time, but at least the seed had been planted.

Living in New York City in the 1970's, I discovered Seth, a non-physical entity who dictated a series of remarkable books through a humble, unassuming medium by the name of Jane Roberts. The flagship of the series, "The Nature of Personal Reality," bears the message: "What we believe will be our reality." I'm still of the opinion this may be the most important book ever written.

Throughout my life, I'd read numerous books with similar messages like "Psycho Cybernetics" by Maxwell Maltz and "Think and Grow Rich," by Napoleon Hill.

Then I was introduced to Abraham, another non-physical entity who speaks through Esther Hicks. Their many books, tapes, and videos are based on the "Law of Attraction" which says, "We get what we focus on." I get daily emails from the Abraham-Hicks website, and find them helpful in keeping my mind on track... in other words, focused on what I want rather than what I don't want.

Abraham says that all anyone really wants is to feel good; that everything we do—accumulating wealth, prestige, accomplishments, losing weight, getting healthy, being of service, etcetera—is ultimately for the purpose of feeling better whether we realize it or not. Abraham suggests finding and focusing on the thoughts that make us feel better; if we'll just do that, everything else will fall into place. That is, we'll get all the money, success, and good health that we need because we'll be thinking in the right direction.

Now even if you don't believe in non-physical entities (spirits?) the practice of focusing on what makes us feel better is not bad advice if you ask me.

All these books and teachings send the same message, and that is, I must take charge of my mind, because what I think about most is what I will end up experiencing.

Gandhi said, "Be the change you want." Does it get any simpler than that? He rallied millions and conquered one of the most powerful nations on the planet without firing a shot—by focusing on what he (and his fellow countrymen) wanted; by stubbornly holding that vision in his mind until he achieved success. Of course, he did a lot of walking while he was at it.

Even the fountainhead of Christianity is quoted as saying, "Ask and you shall receive." It's a different way of saying the same thing. We get what we think about. Thinking about something, especially really focusing on something, is a way of asking for it whether we want it or not.

Some say this is magical thinking, and not based in reality. But what is reality?

The ancient Hindus tell us reality is an illusion. Modern day physicists hint at the same possibility. In 1975, Fritjof Capra published "The Tao of Physics" which I would call a forerunner to modern day quantum physics. In this classic, he describes what is found in sub-nuclear realms. He said we keep looking deeper and deeper into the makeup of matter, and we can't seem to find any truly finite particles. He says every time we discover a very small, sub-nuclear particle, we take a closer look and discover it's not really a particle at all, but an even smaller particle vibrating so fast as to create the illusion of being a solid object. Think of an airplane propeller spinning so fast is looks like a solid disc.

I've heard astrophysicists say the more we understand the universe, the more it's looking like one, big, Virtual Reality software program—all composed of electrical energy!

Quantum Mechanics implies nothing exists unless there is someone to observe it. Remember the age old question: If a tree falls in the woods, and there's no one around to hear it, does it really make any sound? There are still those who dismiss Quantum Physics, but all through history, the truly revolutionary sciences have initially been rejected. We don't like to abandoned our hard-earned beliefs.

Still, the ancient Hindu scriptures and modern day physics suggest essentially the same thing... we live in a dream. There's nothing really here. It's all in our heads. Not to say the dream doesn't seem real. It seems very real indeed. If I hit my thumb with a hammer, it's going to hurt like hell. But then we've been dreaming a very long time... conceivably since the instant of Creation.

"Reality is merely an illusion, albeit a very persistent one."
~ Albert Einstein

I don't want to get too esoteric, so let's look at a more down-to-earth example. Envision a ghetto. The kids grow up surrounded by drugs and violence, right? That's the reality they're faced with, and that's what most of them end up focusing on. To them, it's a matter of survival. But why is it a few of these kids can break free from that reality and end up going to Yale Medical School like the legendary Dr. Ben Carson? Ben grew up poor with learning disabilities, and became a world-renowned neurosurgeon.

George Lopez, Denzel Washington, Will Smith, Martin Luther King, just to name a few, all grew up in less than favorable environments, yet went on to being successful and making a positive difference in the world. I suspect they all had someone in their lives, a parent or some other mentor, who taught them they could do anything they wanted to do if only they would focus their minds... focus on what they wanted, that is, rather than what they saw all around them. This involves discipline. This means conquering the mind. Left to its own devices, the mind will run astray like an untrained mutt, stopping to sniff every pile of dung it comes across.

Dr. John Sarno's wonderful book, "The Mind-Body Connection," suggests that essentially all disease is psychosomatic, i.e. originates in the mind. Do yourself a favor... read it. If you have back problems, read his classic, "Healing Back Pain." I suffered terrible lower back pain for years even after visiting numerous chiropractors. My pain disappeared permanently before I even finished John Sarno's book. Abraham, by the way, *insists* that all disease is psychosomatic.

When I was first diagnosed with cancer, I found another book that became my bible for recovery: "Getting Well Again" by the husband and wife oncology team, Dr. Carl Simonton and his wife, Stephanie.

In documenting their 20 years of experience dealing with cancer victims, they noted a trend: virtually all of their patients had suffered some kind of childhood trauma which seriously damaged their sense of self-esteem. They ended up sub-consciously recreating similar difficulties in their adult lives in order to reaffirm their deeply embedded (false) belief that they lacked self-worth. They did this to the extent they finally reached a point of utter hopelessness. Mentally, they threw in the towel. Sending this message to their bodies, their immune systems collapsed, and the cancer (lying dormant in almost all of us) was given free rein to wreak havoc.

The reason "Getting Well Again" became my "bible" was because I identified with this pattern completely. As a boy, I'd bought into, or believed, my father's constant suggestions that I was unworthy. I subconsciously carried this into adult life. I gravitated toward a very tough business that told me—for many, many years— that I was no good, my movie scripts weren't good enough. I lived in a state of chronic stress. What was I going to do if I didn't make it? How would I survive as an old man? Would I die penniless on the streets? Despite my determination, I finally reached a point of hopelessness and psychologically threw in the towel. I remember exactly when it occurred. After working my tail off all those years, an event led me to believe I was finally on the verge of a major break-though. But the deal fell apart. I was crushed, devastated, more so than I'd ever been. Three months later, I was diagnosed.

By simply helping their patients recognize their repressed, self-destructive modus operandi and restore a sense of worthiness, the Simontons were able to cure even Stage Four cancer patients, achieving a recovery rate more than double that of the national average. Imagine! Curing Stage Four cancer by changing one's mental outlook! I should note this method was not a substitute for conventional treatment, but rather a supplement. Not bad considering the rest of the medical establishment had written these folks off.

I'd like to mention a classic book I recently rediscovered: "The 7 Habits of Highly Successful People" by Sephen R. Covey. Though he's coming from the perspective of solving personal and professional problems, he emphasizes that taking responsibility for your state of mind is your first priority. My personal summary of his 7 habits is as follows:

• Be responsible for your STATE OF MIND

• Know your ULTIMATE PURPOSE in life

• Always make your ultimate purpose your 1st PRIORITY

• Always work for the WIN-WIN agreement

• Honestly empathize, THEN negotiate

• SYNERGIZE–Allow, Integrate, Balance

• FOREVER IMPROVE physically, mentally, spiritually, socially

I highly recommend this book for anyone.

HEALING

But if personal beliefs affect our reality, why is it so many of us experience similar things? Is it because there is a "true" reality? In my opinion, not exactly. Seth explains we exist within a "herd belief system." In other words, what the masses of people believe becomes a "reality" in and of itself. For example, if we can manifest whatever we want by thinking about it, why can't a person grow back an arm that's been cut off? I contend that since so many humans have believed, for so long, that it's not possible to grow back a limb, that herd belief is so powerful it's almost impossible for any of us to break free from it. And yet there are animals who can grow back their limbs.

That brings up another important concept: I personally believe that just about anything can be healed. I just have to BELIEVE I can heal, and I have to WANT to heal. The world is full of examples of people who've defied medical "belief," and recovered from the impossible. It's all about belief and focus.

After receiving external radiation treatment to kill the cancer in my prostate, my radiologist decided I needed radioactive seed implants as well. After all, I had this extremely rare, highly aggressive type of cancer that was known to be a die-hard. Within twenty-four hours of having the radioactive seeds (ninety-four of them) inserted into my prostate, my urethra swelled up so much, I couldn't urinate. Yikes!

If you've ever not been able to pee, you know it's got to be one of the most painful experiences known to man or woman. My wife had to rush me to the emergency room in the middle of the night. I ended up needing a super-pubic catheter for a little over a year in order to relieve my bladder. When the catheter was finally removed, I went from not being able to urinate to becoming completely incontinent! OMG! I'm too young for this, I thought.

Essentially, all that radiation fried the valves that control the release of urine, and almost everything around them. My prostate was reduced to a flap of leather, and my drainage system was a wilted mass of damaged pipeline. My urologist shrugged his shoulders and basically told me, "Shit happens. There's not much we can do."

I researched the issue. I discovered many other men who'd been left in the same predicament, all believing they were simply stuck for life wearing diapers and catheters. But I knew I could... and would heal. I simply believed and allowed my body to do its work. I'm happy... VERY happy to report that everything is finally working just fine now. No diapers or catheters for this camper. Even the frequent urges to go have at last dissipated. I could have easily bought into the belief that I was screwed for life which would have put a damper on, and maybe even prevented my healing. But fortunately, I not only knew I could heal, but had undergone enough personal healing experiences in my life to believe it with my heart and soul. I had to ignore the naysayers, and have faith, patience, and perseverance. I had to direct my thoughts daily with a confident smile on my face.

So once again, we see the necessity of disciplining the mind. Am I going to believe in hopelessness just because everyone else does? Like those kids in the ghettos who believe they're trapped in a world of drugs and violence and there is simply no way out? Or can I stand alone, and choose to believe something else like Dr. Ben Carson who broke out of his immediate herd belief system, and formed a very personal and positive one of his own?

I know, without question, that I MUST take control of my thoughts, and focus on what I want rather than what I don't want. I've learned this the hard way. I also know, that if I ever slip back into hopelessness, the cancer is lying in wait, and is perfectly capable of rearing its ugly head again. I'd rather not go that way.

Thinking positive and focusing on the solution rather than the problem is not always easy at first. It takes work, practice, and determination. Often our minds—because of our egos—tend to focus on fear. It's my ego's job to keep me alive. If I give my ego too much power, it will find things to worry about no matter where I look. That way the ego can feel important. It can say, "Look. I've kept you alive, out of danger, by pointing out all these threats. You need to place me on a pedestal, and worship me like a god. I'm in charge!"

NOT. By focusing on fear, I will only gravitate toward the thing I'm fearing. The ego has its job, but I mustn't give it too much importance. I must keep it in check. Guidance from what I call my Higher Power takes precedence over anything else. More on Higher Power later.

I've learned a couple of practices that help me more than anything else to manage stress, stay out of fear, and focus on the positive:

1 -- Letting Go
2 -- Living in the Moment

LETTING GO

For years I attended a meditation class. Our instructor taught us many things, but the one theme that kept repeating was that of "Letting Go." Letting go means not holding on to resentments, or fears, or angers, or grudges. It often entails forgiving someone or myself. By hating someone for what they did to me hurts me far more than that person.

Often times the best way to love a person is to ALLOW them to be as they are; not try to change them; let go of my own beliefs about how they should behave. There's a reason we live in a world of variety. It's supposed to be that way. Loving and Allowing are really the same thing. Surely you've heard the saying, "If you love someone, let them go."

Sometimes letting goes means releasing something that I really, really want. Because I have an obsessive nature, I can want something too much! It means I'm holding on to it so tightly it doesn't have a chance to grow, to manifest.

There's a saying in Alcoholic's Anonymous: "Let go, let God." In order to grow a plant, I have to put it in the ground, cover it up, water it, and otherwise leave it be. If I keep digging it up to see if it's growing, it never will. Same with manifesting our desires. If I cling too tightly, they won't have a chance to materialize. I need to turn them over to a Power Greater Than Myself. I call that Power, simply, The Universe.

By the way, I do believe in God. What I don't believe are the definitions of God that men have come up with over the ages. I just can't find a suitable one; don't believe it's possible, really. And I've spent my entire life searching. So I tend to use words like "Universe" instead, or "Higher Power." This is a personal preference and just feels better to me. I think we each have to find our own path to "The Source" or "Creator."

I know one thing—the Universe (and now science suspects there may be an infinite number of them) is way more mysterious than we can ever know. Its secrets unfold daily and will always continue to do so. Personally, I'm wary of people who claim to have figured it all out. They're probably just after the green stuff inside my wallet. Having said that... to each his own.

To Let Go means surrendering and having faith that the Universe knows what it's doing. After all, it's been doing a pretty good job of MANIFESTING FROM NOTHING for over 15 billion years now, right? And if you believe that God created everything, then He, too, created from nothing, did He not?

LIVING IN THE MOMENT

Letting Go and Living in the Moment go hand in hand. If I can focus on the right here and now, I'm letting go of the past and the future. Living in the moment means I'm not fretting about that unpleasant thing that happened this morning. Nor am I worrying about that terrible thing that may or may not happen tomorrow. It's been my experience that 99.999% of the time, this present moment is perfectly fine! If I'm feeling uncomfortable, it's almost always because I'm torturing myself about a past event, or worrying about the future.

In his seminal book, "The Power of Now," Eckhart Tolle tells us there is only the Eternal Now. Everything else is either the past or the future which only exists in the mind. He suggests simple techniques like counting your footsteps when going up or down the stairs in order to practice living in the Now. Or paying attention to your breathing. And it does take practice. I've been practicing for almost ten years, and I still haven't mastered it... but I've sure gotten better at it!

Seth tells us that our Point of Power (to change anything) is always in the Present.

MEDITATION

I've been practicing mediation for a very long time. For me, meditation has come to mean intimately connecting with my Higher Power. Again, I don't know exactly what this Higher Power is, or how to explain it, but I know it exists. Whether we call it God, Universe, Spirit, Higher Consciousness, or Source Energy... even if you're an atheist, you've got to admit there is probably something greater than yourself out there... or deep within.

When I meditate, I go within. Every night just before I go to sleep, and every morning as soon as I wake up, I meditate for fifteen minutes. The practice is really very simple: Find a quiet spot and get in a comfortable position. You don't have to sit Lotus style, you just need to be relaxed and comfortable (but not so much that you fall asleep.) Sit up straight. I light two candles, shove my pillows up against my headboard, and sit Indian style. Concentrate on relaxing all the muscles in your body from head to toe. Next, slow your breathing. Take slow, deep breaths. You will notice by slowing your breathing, you slow down the thoughts in your head.

Meanwhile, don't worry about your thoughts. Just let them flow. But if you find yourself holding on to a particular thought, just let it go. At first you'll keep grabbing and holding onto thoughts. You'll assess them, engage with them, multiply them. You'll mold them like clay. Just keep letting them go again, over and over and over. After awhile, you'll get into the habit of doing it automatically and you'll be able to clear your mind.

If you meditate at night, you'll want to let go of all the "stuff" that happened that day. If you meditate in the morning, you want to clear all the "stuff" you wrestled with in your sleep, and start the day with a fresh, clean slate.

Sit still, slow your breathing, and LET GO. That's all it is. Kids do this naturally. Ever see a child staring wide-eyed into space? With a slight grin on his face? He/she is meditating! They know instinctively they have to let go of the thought process now and then in order to allow their Higher Consciousness to analyze their situation and come up with the best solutions for their problems.

I have learned the portal or connection to my Higher Power is in my Heart. After getting very still and emptying my mind, I reside in my heart chakra. There, I imagine a doorway filled with light. I OPEN my chakra by letting go of all my fears, and allowing that light to come out and engulf my entire being, in fact my entire world. That light is Universal Love, the most powerful healing force there is. It keeps the whole universe balanced in a state of exquisite harmony.

When I was a young man living in New York City, I met a Tibetan monk. He taught a group of us what he called "true transcendental meditation." He said if anyone ever charges you money to learn transcendental meditation, it wasn't *true* transcendental meditation. What he taught is pretty much what I just described above. But he added another element... color. He taught us how to heal ourselves by meditating, then imagining our bodies— particularly the part of our bodies that was out of balance—engulfed in violet light. He said hold this vision for as long as possible.

I've used this technique to heal myself and others on several occasions. Remarkably, I once used it to grow enamel back on my teeth, something a dentist will tell you is impossible.

Don't be afraid of Magical Thinking. The world is more malleable than we think. It's simply made of energy—this subtle, ephemeral substance that is intelligent and alive. I believe it responds to our very thoughts.

"Your thoughts shape you." Albert Einstein

Speaking of thoughts, one last one... sometimes, no matter what we do, or what we think about or focus on; no matter how hard we try to heal or manifest, it just won't happen. I've come to believe this can occur primarily because our spirit or Higher Self has its own agenda—an agenda that is, more often than not, beyond our comprehension. When this happens, I have no choice but to stop fighting, and surrender or let go. The results are inevitably for the best in the long run.

There might be other elements standing in the way of a goal as well. Technically, this discussion could fall under the category of stress management, but somehow I'm compelled to give it its own chapter.

CHAPTER SUMMARY

Arguably the most important skill I can ever learn is the ability to direct my thoughts. By focusing on what I want, rather than what I don't want; the solution rather than the problem; by allowing, and living in the moment, I will reduce stress, keep my immune system strong, and remain healthy.

CHAPTER FOUR
EXTRANEOUS INFLUENCES

"Mama always said, life is like a box of chocolates. You never know what you're gonna get."
~ Forrest Gump

Not long ago, I went on a ten mile hike into the California Big Sur wilderness. I traversed a variety of terrain. The trail went up, and the trail went down. There were stretches where the Poison Oak grew so close on either side, I had to carefully pick my way through to avoid touching it. There were sections of cool, forest shade, and stretches of open space and blazing heat. I was chased by crazed flies, and enjoyed moments of peace and beauty. The hike was a lot of work, but I came back to camp that evening feeling exhilarated... with a sense of accomplishment. I'd had an adventure. It has been said we are spirits on a human adventure.

On the drive home back to Santa Barbara, I realized life is like that trail hike—always changing—and I just have to adapt. I have another analogy for life: Life is like being in a boat out in the ocean. Most of the time, the water is calm and the skies clear. But sometimes a storm will hit, and all we can do is hang on for dear life.

What's interesting is, this seems to be true even if I never leave my house! Sometimes, I'm feeling perfectly fine, and sometimes bothered. Often, I don't even know why. But these changes in being are almost always a result of what's going on in my head. But are there factors that influence what comes up in my head? Factors beyond what I purposely focus on?

I suspect so. Think of this... here we are, living on this tiny earthen orb, racing through the cosmos at an unfathomable speed, passing through all kinds of invisible fields—radio waves, gamma rays, electromagnetic fields, gravitational fields, solar flares, gases, vacuums, all sorts of inexplicable radiation zones, and God only knows what else! We've got to be affected by these things, and not even realize it. Can these things affect my moods? Even my health?

Then, of course, we have to consider the fact that the brain is constantly manufacturing chemicals that affect our mental outlook. Foods can change our chemical makeup. Did you know that when you smile, your brain creates Seratonin, a chemical which makes you feel better? Go ahead, try it. Make yourself smile whether you feel like it or not. I mean a BIG smile. Hold it for at least 15 seconds, and I'll bet you'll end up laughing for no reason. And when you go into a state of stress or fear, your body creates other chemicals that can definitely create the opposite feeling.

If we're all psychic (or intuitive) to some degree or another, what about all those brain waves I might be picking up from other people? Why do I suddenly hear old songs in my head? Am I some kind of human radio?

Astrology has long been a hobby of mine. I favor the ancient Hindu astrology, otherwise known as Vedic Astrology, which is considered a Sacred Science. Thousands of years ago, men realized the moon influences bodies of water causing the ebb and flow of tides. They noted that their crops were also influenced by the moon, and discovered the best times to plant and harvest.

It's not too much of a stretch to realize that if the moon has some kind of mysterious, gravitational pull that can affect entire oceans, what about all those other stars and planets out there with their influences?

Thus astrology was born. But since it involves invisible forces, immeasurable by instruments, it's not accepted as "science" per se. But to me, it's a no brainer: If the moon can tug something as massive as an ocean, what can it do to the chemicals in my brain?

So these ancient Hindus started documenting what they observed. They made careful notes, generation after generation, about the similarities they saw during different alignments of the sun, moon, planets, and stars. After doing this for many centuries, they saw the same patterns repeated over and over and over. Hence they were able to make some predictions based on when a person was born and what cosmic forces were influencing him during his lifetime. Did you know that countless kings, queens, presidents, and celebrities have consulted astrologers over the ages?

Besides the influences of bodies in space, we have Biorhythms, again not an official "science," but still somewhat compelling. If women can go through menstrual cycles, can't men go through something similar? At times, it certainly feels like it to me.

Then there's the subject of dimensions. M-Theory, a division of theoretical physics, postulates there are at least seven other dimensions in order for the four we accept (the fourth being time) to even exist. That's a total of eleven dimensions we believe must exist just for us to be here. How many more will we discover? Who knows what subtle, invisible forces we're immersed in, affecting us on myriad levels, yet we're completely unaware of them.

Lastly, as mentioned at the end of the last chapter, there's my soul's agenda. Conceivably, my spirit or Higher Self, has a much smarter plan for me than I do, especially if it is a timeless, all-knowing entity (which, of course, I can't prove). Nonetheless, it's important for me to remember this. So often, I think I know what's best for me, only to be stopped in my tracks. I've resisted enough in my life to know it's sometimes futile to keep struggling. More often than not, if I really push, or force, my own agenda, it backfires. Then again fighting Nazis in a world war is another story. Thankfully, I don't have to fight any wars except the ones in my head. Normally, I've learned if something doesn't unfold following a path of least resistance, it doesn't work out well. I've learned to surrender DAILY to my Higher Power. In fact, this is part of my morning meditation ritual.

For me, it all boils down to this: We've gotta roll with the punches. Everyone will acknowledge life has its ups and downs. We can't fight it, folks. Roll with it. As Eckhart Tolle says in the beginning of his book, "The Power of Now," he heard a voice that launched his journey of self-discovery. That voice said simply, "Resist nothing."

Abraham says stress comes from resistance to what is. Accept what is, then focus on desire. Stress weakens the immune system. When the immune system is weak, disease can set in.

I stopped watching the news, and stopped engaging in politics. Call me un-American, I don't care. I find politics divisive at a time when the world needs to work in harmony. The news magnates have figured out that by blowing things way out of proportion, they can get people hooked on the drama. As far as I'm concerned most news is a distortion of the truth for the purpose of making money (selling advertising) at our expense. They'll have you think the entire planet is in a state of turmoil and despair. And when we all buy into that, guess what... it only makes the problems worse. The best thing I can do is find my own joy and inner peace. Maybe the guy next to me will take note and want some of that. Maybe the best way to change the world is one person at a time.

For me, the notions of surrender, letting go, allowing, loving, and living in the moment are the most important lessons in my life; the most important things I need to practice and master.

I have to trust that some kind of Higher Power will guide me if I'll only let it. That Higher Power knows a hell of a lot more than I do about how to exist in peace and harmony. And isn't that the path to feeling good?

CHAPTER SUMMARY

The best way to navigate life is to surrender to, and trust in a Higher Power of my own understanding.

CHAPTER FIVE
DAILY ROUTINES FOR LIFE

"The price of success is hard work, dedication to the job at hand, and the determination that whether we win or lose, we have applied the best of ourselves to the task at hand."
~ Vince Lombardi

To once again summarize what we've discussed so far, there are three basic areas that comprise my well-being:

• NUTRITION: My research has led me to believe that an organic, plant-based diet is the healthiest and most nutritious way to eat.

• EXERCISE: I want my body to stay strong and fit. Besides strength, I need fresh oxygen and proper circulation for optimal health. The best way to achieve this is through exercise.

• STRESS MANAGEMENT: Arguably the most important skill I can ever learn is the ability to direct my thoughts. By focusing on what I want, rather than what I don't want; the solution rather than the problem; by allowing, and living in the moment, I will reduce stress, keep my immune system strong, and remain healthy.

All this takes effort and discipline. And I'd like to make something perfectly clear right now: In no way have I mastered these things. I'm a work in progress. I'll never attain perfection. I can only keep making the effort, and by doing so, not only does my life get better, but so do the lives of those around me.

"So much work!" some of you say. It's worth it. But there's only one way we can summon the energy to do it. We've got to Love. We've got to love ourselves, first and foremost. That's the only way I can truly love anyone else. Love life. Love the ground you walk on. Love the stars, the whole universe. Love your God. Love a child, a butterfly, your spouse. Next time you see a snail moving across your driveway, instead of squashing it, get down on your hands and knees, and marvel at this magnificent creature. See how it glides so smoothly, like a galleon sailing the sea, carrying its home on its back, thousands of microscopic muscles rippling in perfect unison, antennae erect guiding its course. Let it go this time. It's just trying to survive... just like you and me. Just like all creatures.

When you wake up in the morning, don't start thinking about all the problems that may face you in the day ahead. Do your meditation. Clear your mind. Allow your Higher Power to create the strategies for navigating the world, then let yourself be guided. Surrender. Open your heart like a flower blossoming in the sunlight. Let the love come out. Instead of making a mental fear list, make a mental gratitude list. Be grateful for your miraculous existence. Just like the humble snail, you are a miracle. Your life is precious, and your contribution to the world is greater than you'll ever know.

Be grateful for your blessings—you have so many if you look for them. Find the thoughts that make you feel good, the ones that put a smile on your face.

Don't get out of bed until you're feeling good. Excited! Make up your mind you're going to pursue your life with passion. Ask your Higher Power to be your partner. Decide to be happy and fearless. Life is short. Make every moment count.

"When you arise in the morning, think of what a precious privilege it is to be alive—to breathe, to think, to enjoy, to love."
~ Marcus Aurelius

Your inner attitude, your perspective, is up to you. It will be reflected in everything around you, inside and out. It always has, and always will be.

(SELECTED) SUGGESTED READING

DIET & RECIPE BOOKS

"**Eat to Live**: The Amazing Nutrient-Rich Program for Fast and Sustained Weight Loss"
Joel Fuhrman, MD

"**Forks Over Knives**: The Plant-Based Way to Health"
Gene Stone, T. Colin Campbell, and Caldwell B. Esselstyn

"**Power Foods for the Brain**"
Neal D. Barnard, MD

"**Prevent and Reverse Heart Disease**: the Revolutionary, Scientifically Proven, Nutrition-Based Cure"
Caldwell B. Esselstyn Jr., M.D.

"**The 150 Healthiest Foods on Earth**: The Surprising, Unbiased Truth About What You Should Eat and Why"
George Mateljan

"**The Bragg Healthy Lifestyle**: Vital Living to 120!"
Paul Bragg and Patricia Bragg

"**The China Study**: The Most Comprehensive Study of Nutrition Ever Conducted And the Startling Implications for Diet, Weight Loss, And Long-term Health"
T. Colin Campbell

"**The Engine 2 Diet**: The Texas Firefighter's 28-Day Save-Your-Life Plan to Lower Cholesterol and Burn Away the Pounds:
Rip Esselstyn

"**The McDougall Program**: 12 Days to Dynamic Health"
John A. McDougall

"**The Millennium Cookbook**: Extraordinary Vegetarian Cuisine"
Eric Tucker, John Westerdahl, Sascha Weiss

"**The New 8-Week Cholesterol Cure**: The Ultimate Program for Preventing Heart Disease"
Robert E. Kowalski

"**The Spectrum**. A scientifically proven program to feel better, live longer, lose weight, gain health"
Dean Ornish, M.D.

"**Medical Medium**: Secrets Behind Chronic and Mystery Illness and How to Finally Heal"
Anthony William

Websites:

"**Bragg Live Food Products**"
www.bragg.com

"**Dr. John Westerdahl**"
www.drwesterdahl.com

"**Nutrition Facts.org**"
www.nutritionfacts.org

"**The Physician's Committee for Responsible Medicine**"
www.pcrm.org

"**The World's Healthiest Foods**"
www.whfoods.com

EXERCISE

"Live Young Forever: 12 Steps to Optimum Health, Fitness, and Longevity"
Jack LaLanne

STRESS (MIND) MANAGEMENT

"Getting Well Again"
O. Carl Simonton, M.D., Stephanie Matthews-Simonton, James L. Creighton

"Healing Back Pain: The Mind-Body Connection"
John E. Sarno M.D.

"Psycho Cybernetics"
Maxwell Maltz

"The 7 Habits of Highly Effective People: Powerful Lessons in Personal Change"
Sephen R. Covey

"The Law of Attraction: The Basics of the Teachings of Abraham"
Esther Hicks and Jerry Hicks

"The Mindbody Prescription: Healing the Body, Healing the Pain"
John E. Sarno M.D.

"The Nature of Personal Reality"
Jane Roberts

"The Power of Now: A Guide to Spiritual Enlightenment"
Eckhart Tolle

"The Power of Positive Thinking"

Norman Vincent Peale

"The Tao of Physics"
Fritjof Capra

"Think & Grow Rich"
Napoleon Hill

Websites:

Abraham-Hicks Publications
www.abraham-hicks.com

ABOUT THE AUTHOR

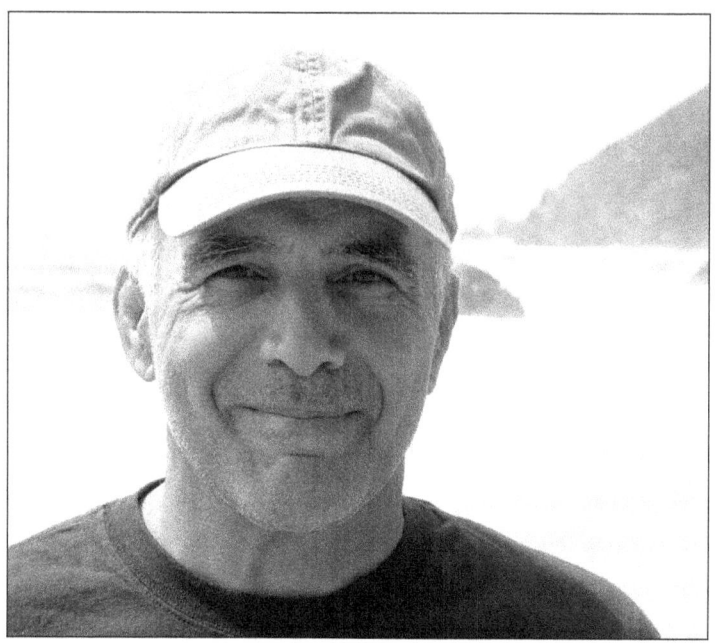

D. A. Metrov

D. A. Metrov is a writer, filmmaker, and fine arts painter. Born and raised in Southern California, he has lived in New York City, Los Angeles, and now resides in Santa Barbara with his wife Maureen and one ornery, black cat. He loves animals, nature, and healthy living.

You may write him at: metrov@lightmasters.net to inquire about speaking and consulting engagements, and bulk book sales. Please leave your review on Amazon.com. Thanks for reading CONQUER THYSELF! Stay healthy and spread the word!